Icy and Refreshing: Infused Water Recipes

Delicious Infused Waters to Keep the Thirst Away

By: Layla Tacy

License Notes

The content of this publication is protected by national and international copyright laws. Hence, you may not reproduce, edit, copy, print, or distribute any part of it, except with express permission of the author.

The author also reserves the right not to be liable for any inference, assumption, or misinterpretation which might lead to any form of damage.

Table of Contents

Introduction

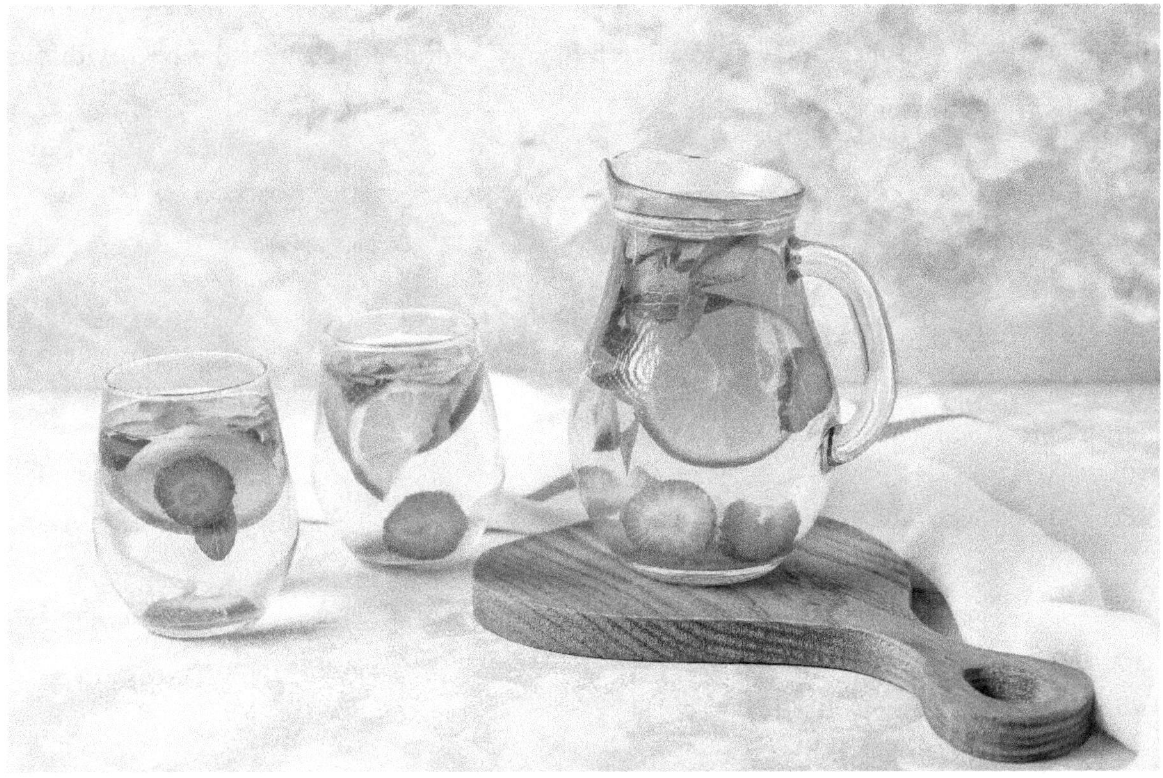

You don't need sodas or juices to quench your thirst on hot days. All you need is some water and fruit. So grab a bottle or pitcher; it doesn't matter, and let's get started! We've already gotten some strawberries, mangos, cherries, nectarines, and more, so let's begin. Besides, what else did you have in mind in order to escape the heat today?

With Icy and Refreshing: Infused Waters, you will learn all of the infusions you need in order to stay hydrated and keep the heat away. You don't need much. As long as you've got water and at least one fruit, we're good to go. Besides, these infusions are also a quick and delicious way to detox while putting all the leftover bits of fruit in your fridge to good use.

While herbs like mint, basil, and rosemary give great flavor to some of our recipes, you'll be happy to hear that they're not 100% necessary. That means if you're looking for a last-minute recipe, but you're all out of herbs, you can enjoy the infusion without them. However, if you want to run to the store and load up on these before we get started, that's fine as well! The point is for you to have fun, stay hydrated, and beat the heat with our delicious fruit infusions. Good luck!

XXXXXXXXXXXXXXXXXXXXXXXXXXXXXXXXXXXXXXXXXXXXXXXXXXXXXXXXXXXXX

Recipe 1: Cherry Infused Water with Ginger

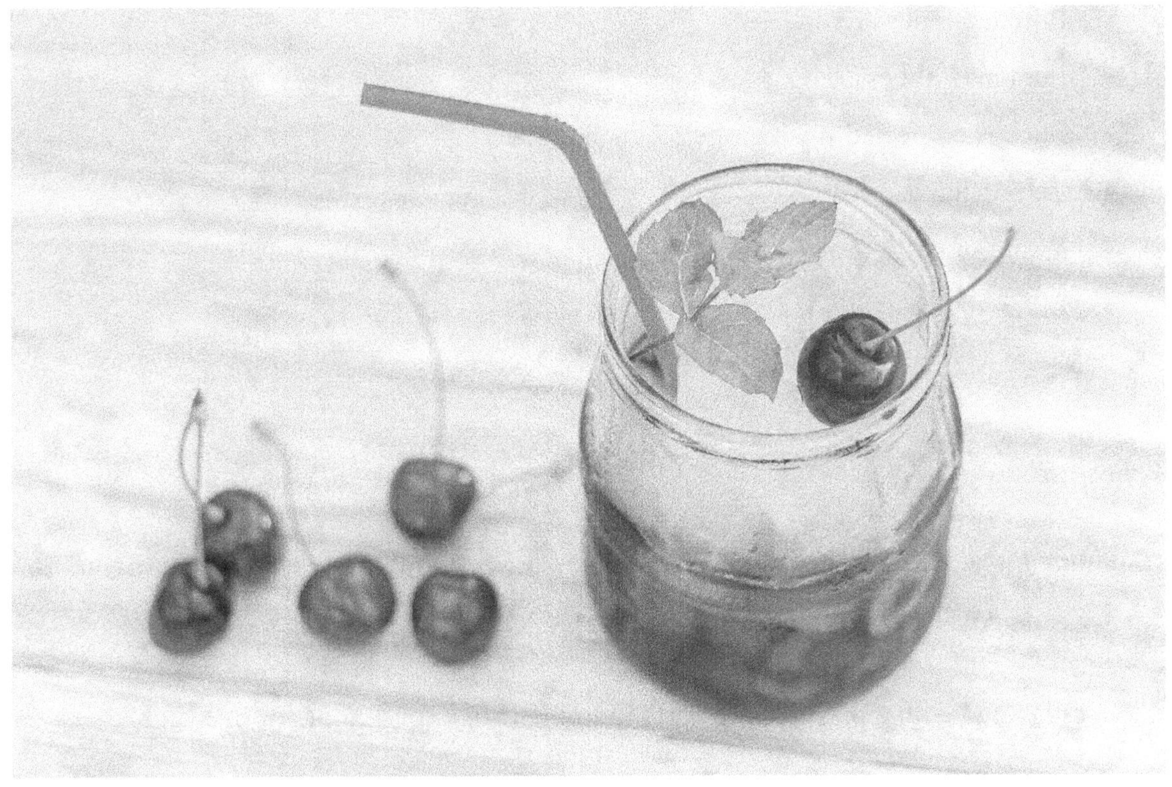

Serving Sizes: 4

Prep Time: 4 hours 15 minutes

Ingredient List:

- Green tea: 4 bags
- Pitted cherries: 1 cup
- Lemon: 4 slices
- Sliced and peeled fresh ginger: 2-inch piece
- Lemon juice: 1 tbsp.
- White sugar: 3 tbsp.
- Filtered water (divided): 4 cups

XXXXXXXXXXXXXXXXXXXXXXXXXXXXXXXXXXXXXXXXXXXXXXXXXXXXXXXXXXXX

Procedure:

Combine ginger slices and cherries in one glass bowl. Sprinkle sugar over the mixture of cherries and cover with filtered water (2 cups).

Cover this bowl with a plastic wrap and put in the fridge for 4 hours or overnight.

Boil two cups filtered water and pour this water over tea bags in one pitcher. Steep tea bags for 90 seconds. Squeeze all tea bags into glass pitcher and discard these bags.

Strain the ginger-cherry water in the glass pitcher with green tea. Squeeze out extra liquid and serve with lemon juice and lemon slices.

Recipe 2: Strawberry Chamomile Infused Water

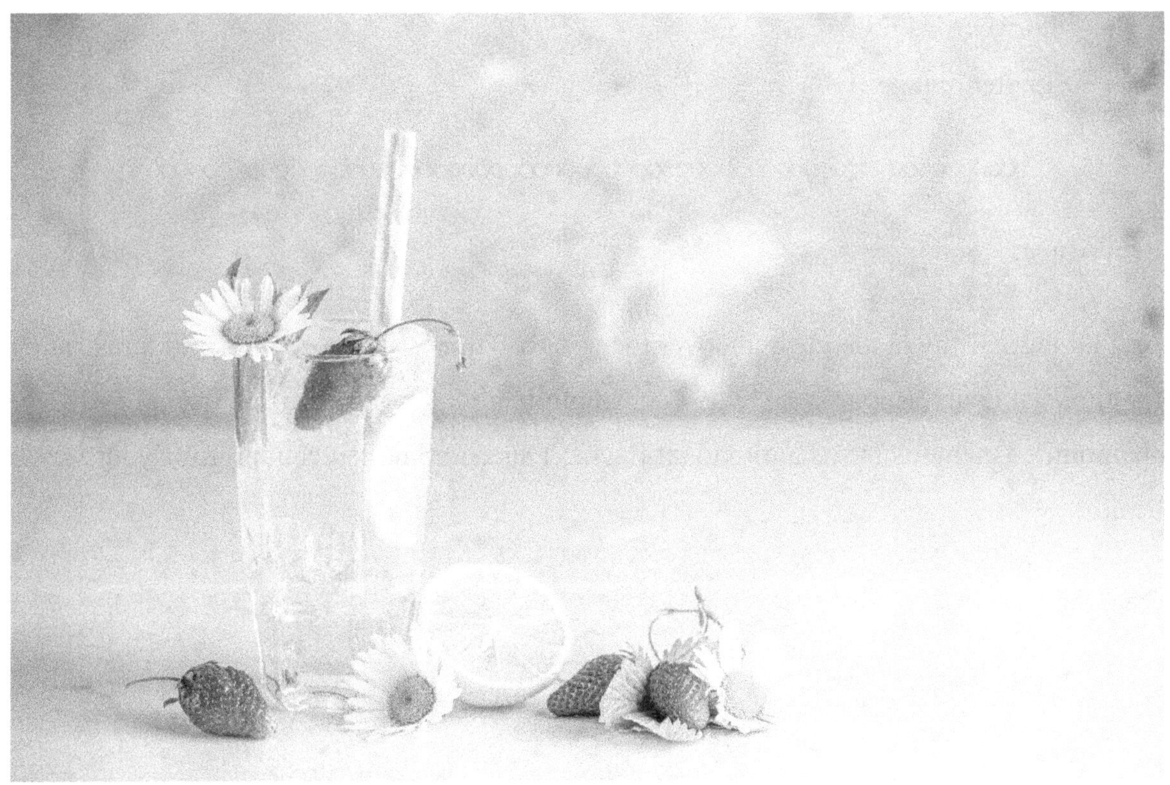

Serving Sizes: 1-liter

Prep Time: 4 hours 10 minutes

Ingredient List:

- Chamomile tea: 1
- Strawberries: 2
- Quarter orange: 1

XXXXXXXXXXXXXXXXXXXXXXXXXXXXXXXXXXXXXXXXXXXXXXXXXXXXXXXXXXXXXX

Procedure:

Add all ingredients in the jug and cover them with 1-liter water. Keep this mixture aside for almost 4 hours. Remove tea bags of chamomile after getting required flavor. The chamomile is famous for its antioxidant flavor. This combination can improve your health.

Recipe 3: Tomato Basil Infusion

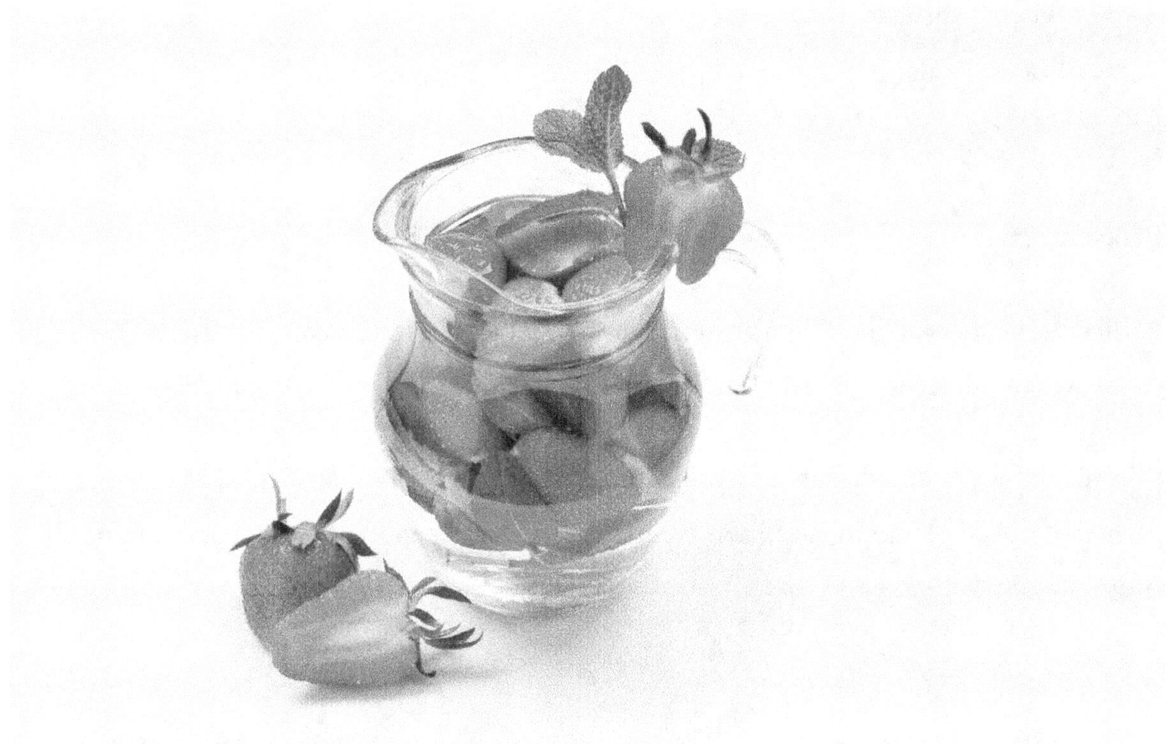

Serving Sizes: 2 quarts

Prep Time: 4 hours 5 minutes

Ingredient List:

- Beefsteak ripe tomato: 1 diced (10 ounces)
- Basil: 3 sprigs
- Water: 2 quarts

XXXXXXXXXXXXXXXXXXXXXXXXXXXXXXXXXXXXXXXXXXXXXXXXXXXXXXXXXXXXXXXX

Procedure:

Pt diced tomatoes and basil sprigs in a glass pitcher. Fill with 2 quarters clean water and cover with a lid. Keep this water in the fridge for 4 hours to infuse all ingredients.

Stir infused water and discard all solids. Serve with fresh sprigs and diced tomatoes for garnishing. Add plenty of ice to serve chilled. You can keep this water secure in your fridge for almost 2 days.

Recipe 4: Hibiscus Infused Water

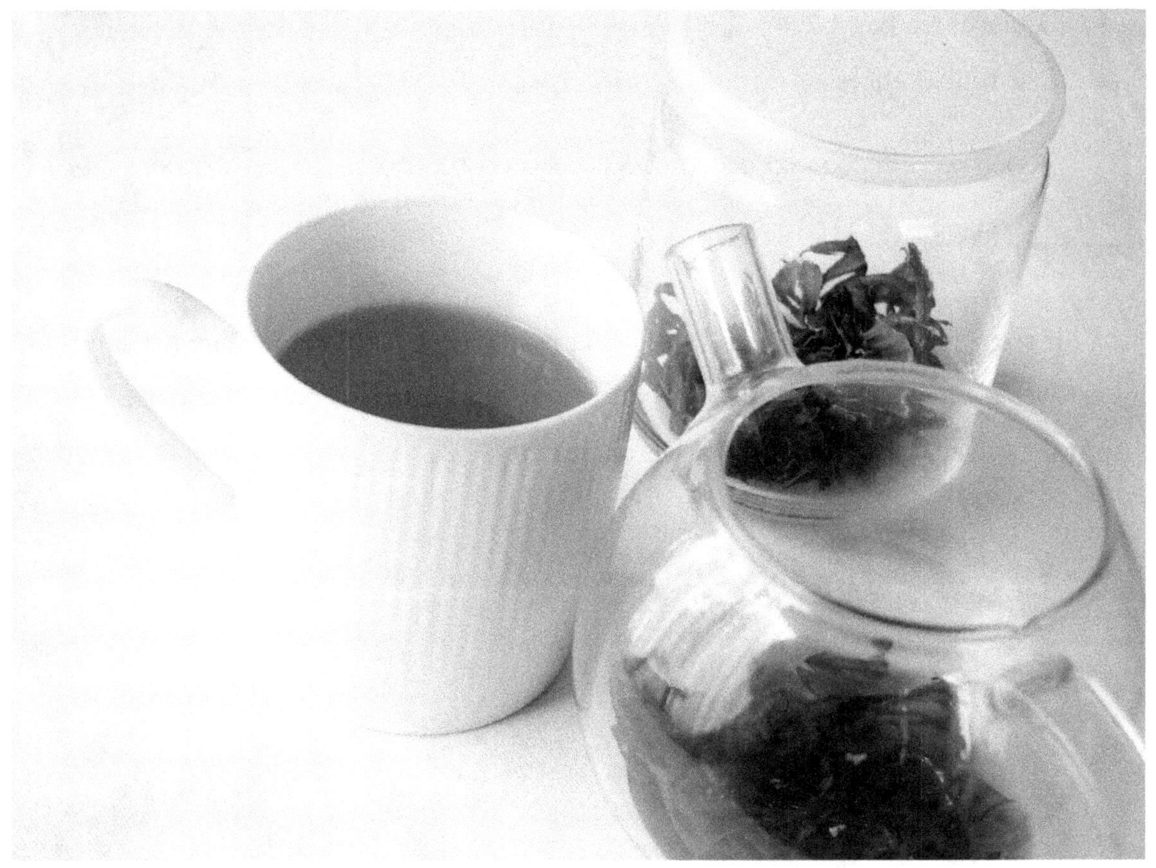

Serving Sizes: 1-liter

Prep Time: 4 hours

Ingredient List:

- Orange: 2 slices
- Hibiscus tea bags: 2
- Star fruit: 3 slices

XXXXXXXXXXXXXXXXXXXXXXXXXXXXXXXXXXXXXXXXXXXXXXXXXXXXXXXXXXXXXX

Procedure:

Put all ingredients in a glass jar and fill this jar with water. Put in the fridge for almost 4 hours to infuse flavors. Drink and enjoy its health benefits. It is good to decrease absorption of sugar and helpful for LDL cholesterol.

Recipe 5: Lime and Blueberry Infusion

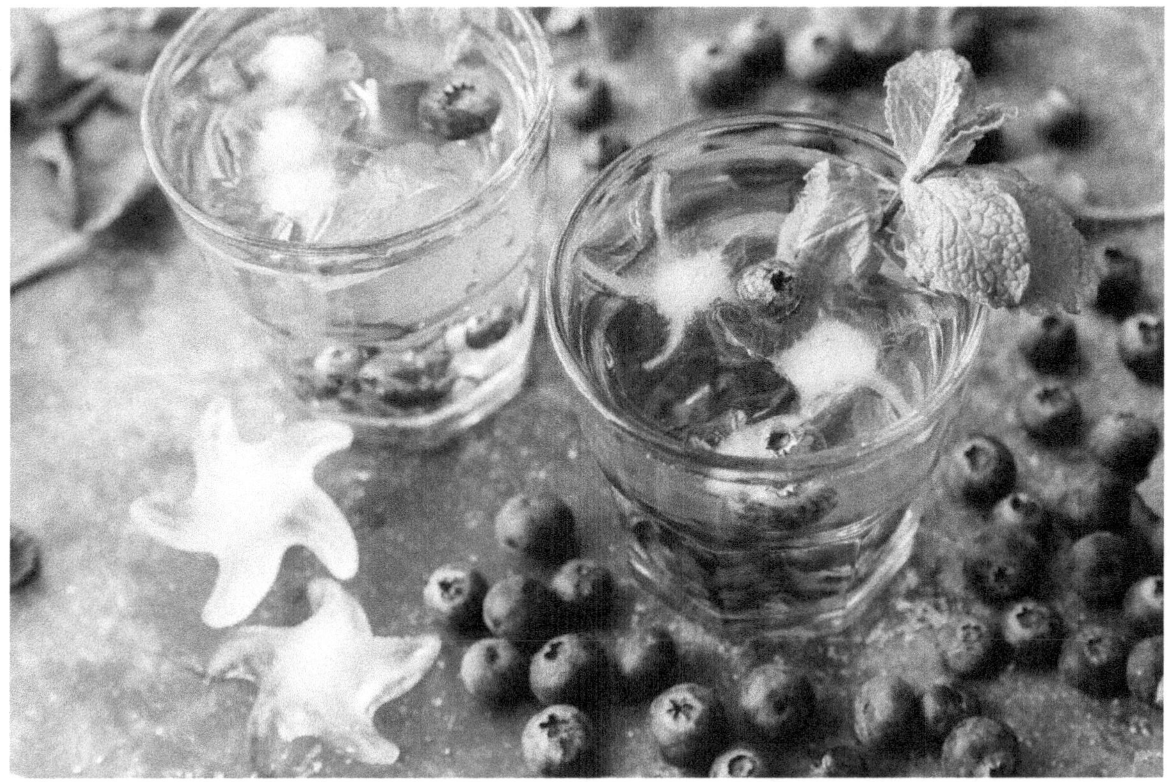

Serving Sizes: 32 ounces

Prep Time: 4 hours

Ingredient List:

- Organic Orange: 2 slices
- Organic lemon: 1 slice
- Blueberries: 8 to 10

XXXXXXXXXXXXXXXXXXXXXXXXXXXXXXXXXXXXXXXXXXXXXXXXXXXXXXXXXXXXXX

Procedure:

Put all ingredients in a glass jar and fill this jar with 32 ounces water. Chill it in the fridge for 4 to 8 hours or 24 hours to infuse maximum flavors. This water can detox your body with its antioxidant properties.

Recipe 6: Cinnamon and Rhubarb Infusion

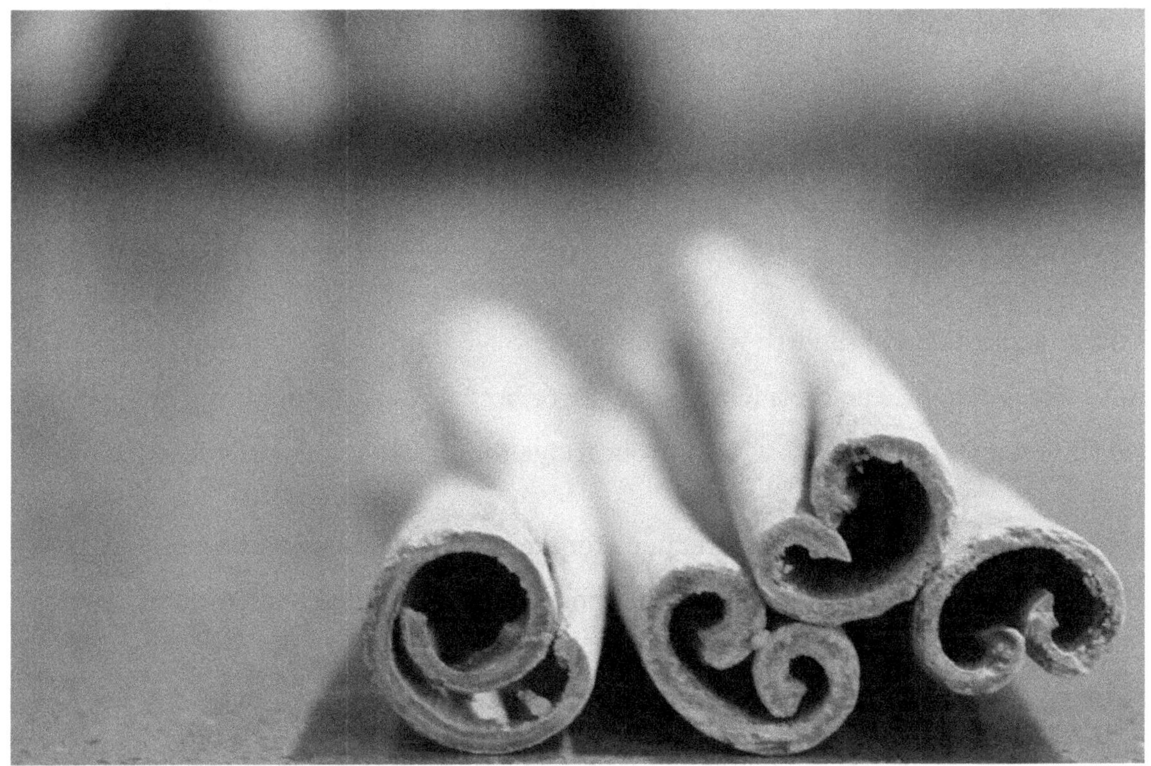

Serving Sizes: 1-liter

Prep Time: 4 hours

Ingredient List:

- Apple: ½
- Cinnamon: 1 stick
- Rhubarb: 1 stick

XXXXXXXXXXXXXXXXXXXXXXXXXXXXXXXXXXXXXXXXXXXXXXXXXXXXXXXXXXXX

Procedure:

Release some juices of rhubarb with your rolling pin before breaking it into small pieces. Make slices of apples before adding it in a jug or bottle. Add all ingredients in the bottle and fill it with water. Put this water in your fridge for almost 4 hours to infuse flavors.

Apples, rhubarb and cinnamon are famous for their nutrient value and fibrous components. These are good to detox your body and provide essential nutrients.

Recipe 7: Green Water

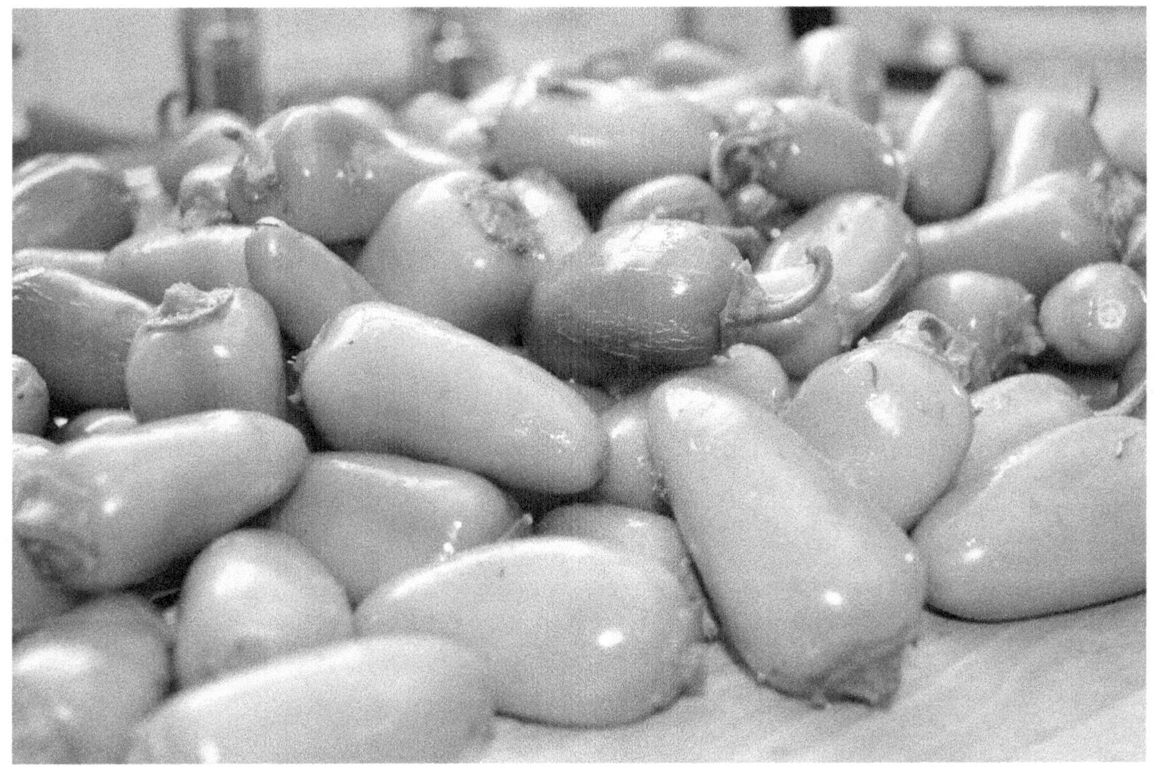

Serving Sizes: 4

Prep Time: 4 hour 5 minutes

Ingredient List:

- Jalapeno pepper: (seeded and halved): 1 large
- Water: 4 cups
- Fresh mint: 2 sprigs
- Cucumber slices: 6 (1/4-inch thick)

XXXXXXXXXXXXXXXXXXXXXXXXXXXXXXXXXXXXXXXXXXXXXXXXXXXXXXXXXXXXXX

Procedure:

Combine mint, jalapeno pepper, cucumber, and water in a glass pitcher. Put in the fridge for almost 4 hours to serve chilled.

Recipe 8: Ginger and Pineapple Infusion

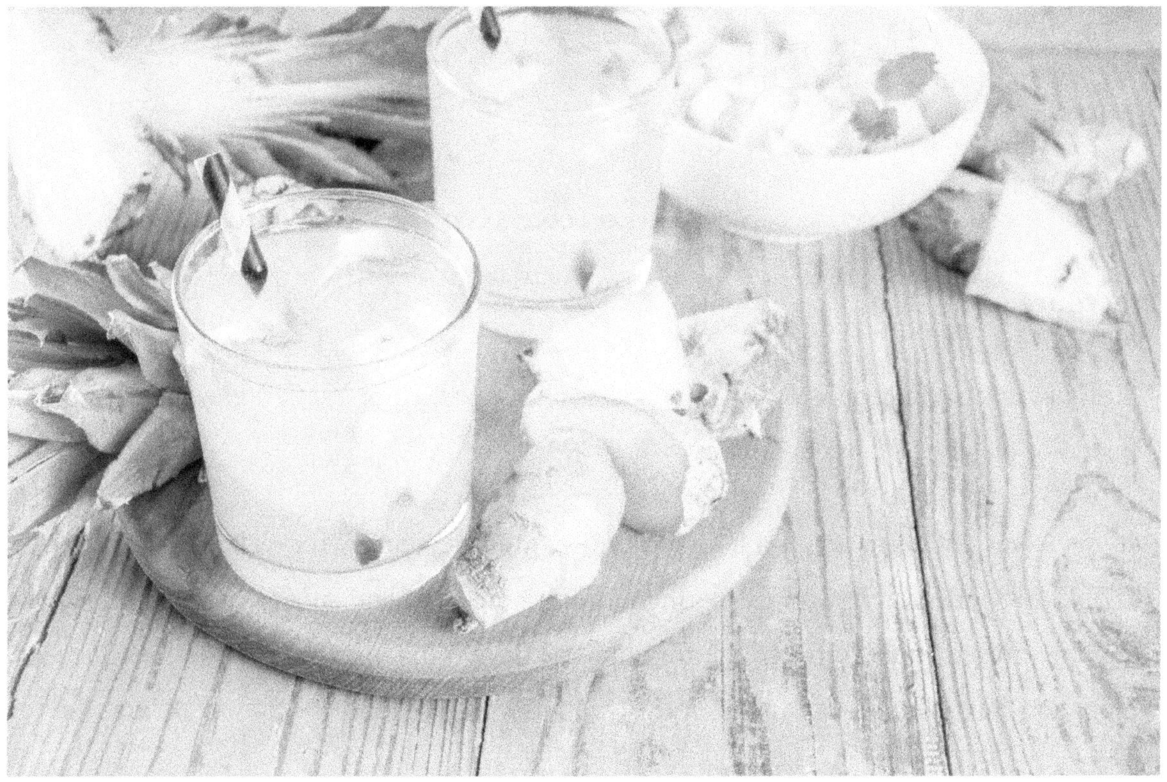

Serving Sizes: 2-quarts

Prep Time: 4 hours 10 minutes

Ingredient List:

- Thin slices of pineapple: 4 cups (almost 1 ¼ pounds)
- Mint: 5 sprigs
- Ginger slices (smashed): 8
- Water: 2-quart

XXXXXXXXXXXXXXXXXXXXXXXXXXXXXXXXXXXXXXXXXXXXXXXXXXXXXXXXXXXX

Procedure:

Add four cups of pineapple slices, mint sprigs and smashed ginger in a glass pitcher. Add 2 quarts of clean water in the pitcher.

Put this water in the fridge for 4 hours to infuse all ingredients. Mix well and strain. You can discard solids. Serve with fresh ginger, mint, pineapple and sufficient ice. You can keep this infused water in the fridge for almost 2 days. This infusion is good to reduce weight and flush toxins out of your body.

Recipe 9: Cucumber Infusion

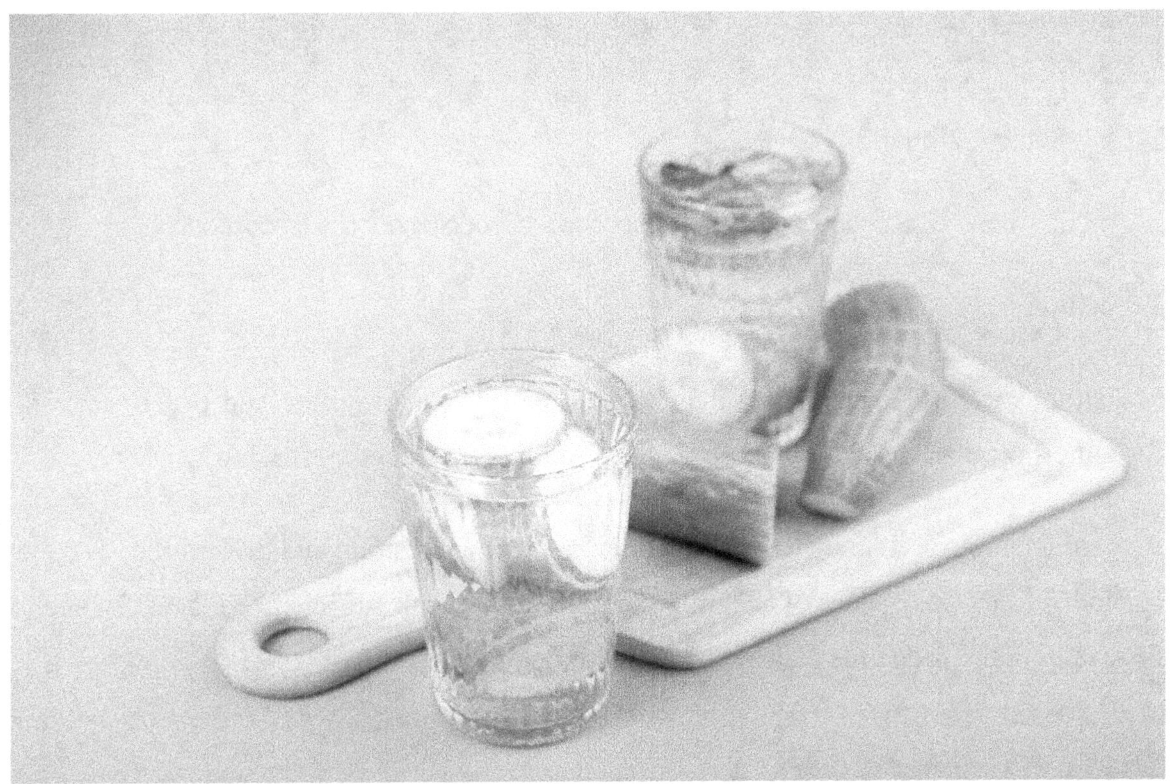

Serving Sizes: 2-quart

Prep Time: 4 hours 5 minutes

Ingredient List:

- English cucumber: 1 (thinly sliced):
- Water: 2-quart
- Ice: as per need
- Seltzer: 2-quart

XXXXXXXXXXXXXXXXXXXXXXXXXXXXXXXXXXXXXXXXXXXXXXXXXXXXXXXXX

Procedure:

Make thin slices of a cucumber and put these slices in 2-quart water. Add 1-quart seltzer for glittering water during preparation. Add second 1-quart before serving.

Put in the fridge for 4 hours to infuse cucumber. Mix well, strain and discard the cucumber. Add fresh slices of cucumber to serve along with sufficient ice. You can keep this water in the fridge for 2 days. It is good to detox your body.

Recipe 10: Citrus Water

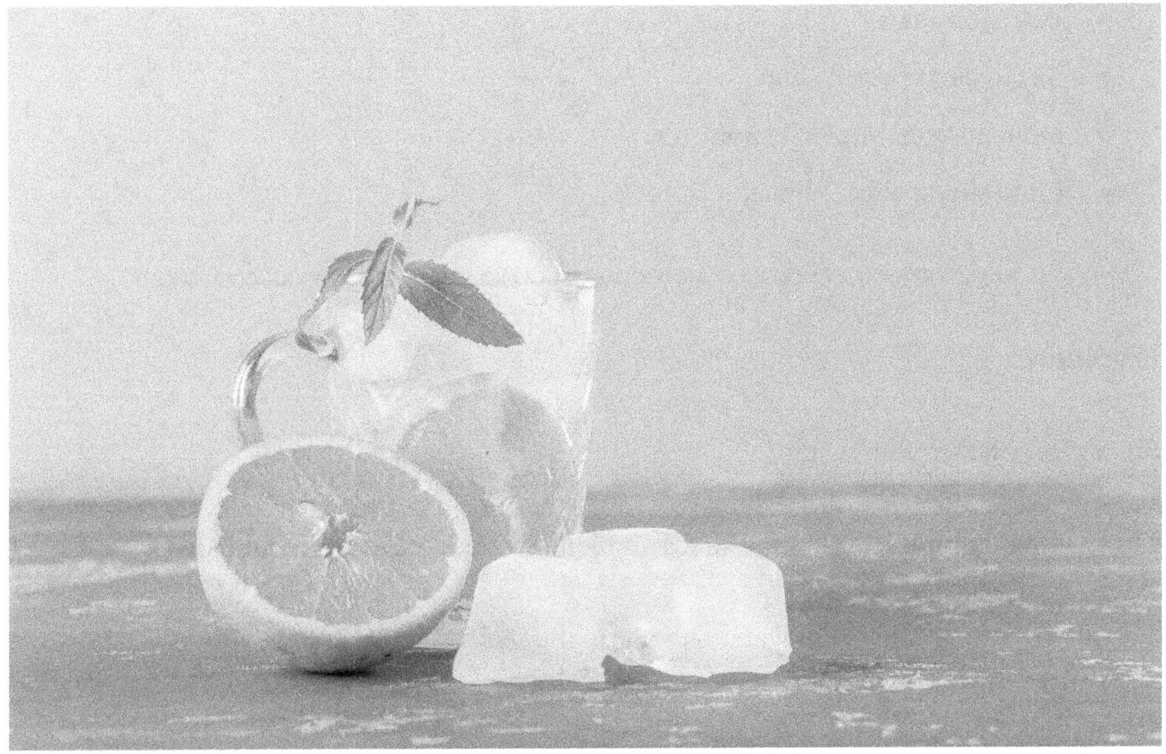

Serving Sizes: 8

Prep Time: 2 days 10 minutes

Ingredient List:

- Mint leaves: ½ cup
- Water: 2-quart
- Sliced cucumber: ½ cup
- Lemon slices: slice 1 lemon
- Lime slices: slice 2 limes

xxxxxxxxxxxxxxxxxxxxxxxxxxxxxxxxxxxxxxxxxxxxxxxxxxxxxxxxxxxxxx

Procedure:

Fill a glass pitcher with water.

Mix cucumber, mint leaves, lime slices and lemon slices together in one bowl.

Add all mixed ingredients in water and put in the fridge for 2 – 3 days. Stir at least once a day to infuse flavors.

Recipe 11: Mint and Mango Infused Water

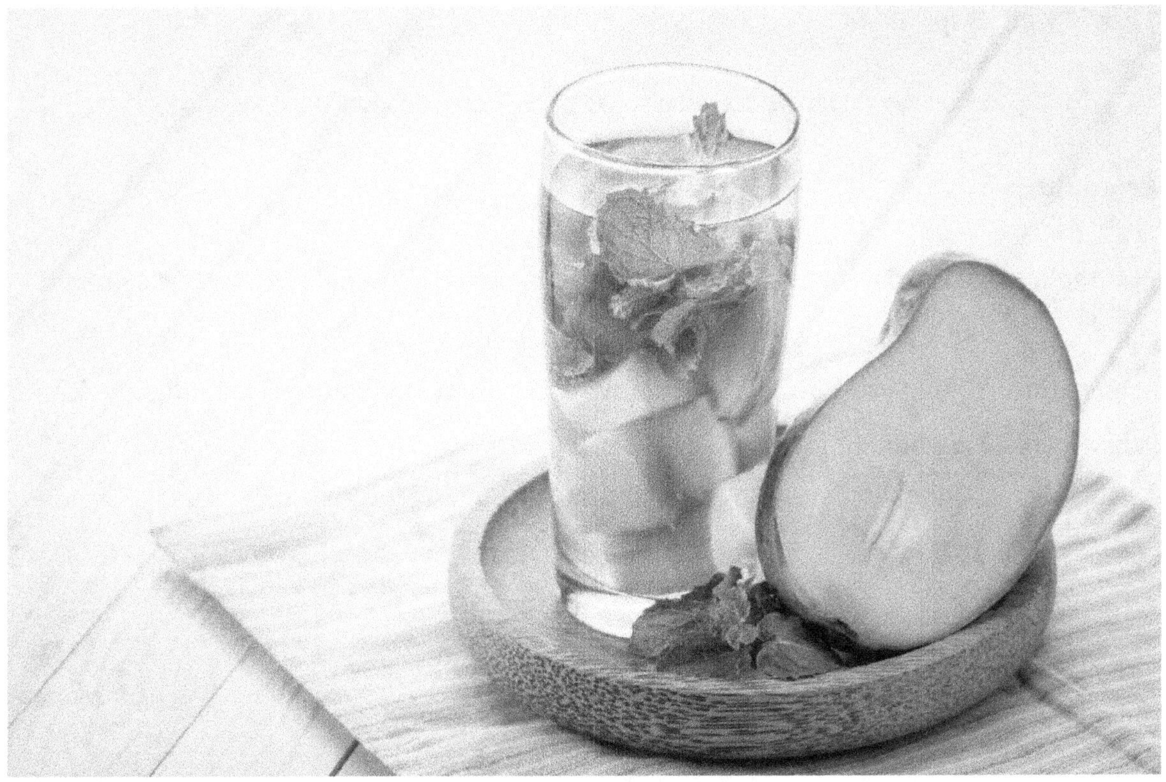

Serving Sizes: 1-liter

Prep Time: 4 hours

Ingredient List:

- Mango: ½
- Mint: 2 sprigs

XXXXXXXXXXXXXXXXXXXXXXXXXXXXXXXXXXXXXXXXXXXXXXXXXXXXXXXXXXXXXX

Procedure:

Peel the mango and cut into six pieces. Add the mango pieces and mint to a Mason jar and cover it with water. Cover the jar and keep it aside for almost 4 hours at room temperature. Mango can infuse in a better way in warm temperature. This infusion drink helps decreasing your cholesterol.

Recipe 12: Herbal Infused Water

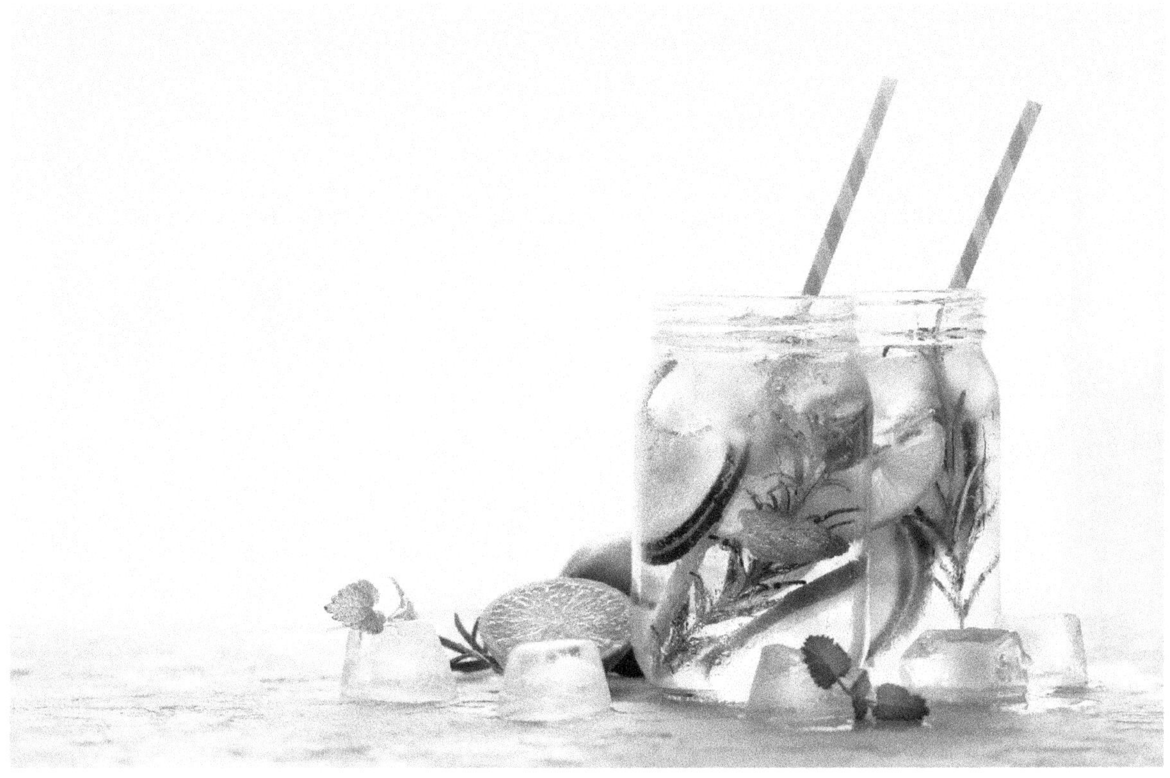

Serving Sizes: 1-liter

Prep Time: 4 hours

Ingredient List:

- Rosemary: 1 sprig
- Dill: 2 sprigs
- Thyme: 1 sprig
- Mint: 2 sprigs

XXXXXXXXXXXXXXXXXXXXXXXXXXXXXXXXXXXXXXXXXXXXXXXXXXXXXXXXXXX

Procedure:

Tear all herb leaves and add in a 1-liter jug. Fill this jug with water and put in the fridge for one night. A healthy herbal and delicious infusion is ready.

Recipe 13: Mint and Watermelon Infusion

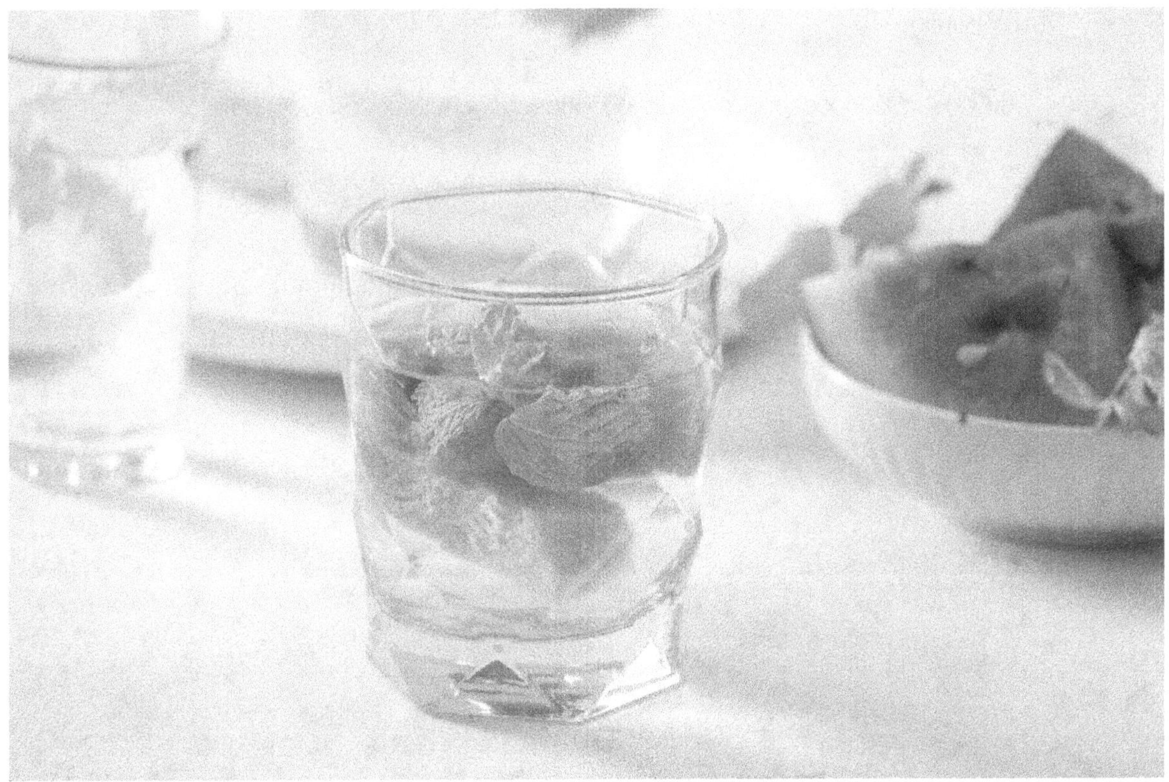

Serving Sizes: 1-liter jar

Prep Time: 4 hours

Ingredient List:

- Watermelon: 1
- Mint: 1 sprig

XXXXXXXXXXXXXXXXXXXXXXXXXXXXXXXXXXXXXXXXXXXXXXXXXXXXXXXX

Procedure:

Chop watermelon into pieces and add in the water. Add all the mint sprigs. Keep it aside for 4 hours or more in the fridge. Serve chilled. It is good to flush all toxins from your body.

Recipe 14: Rosemary Infused Water

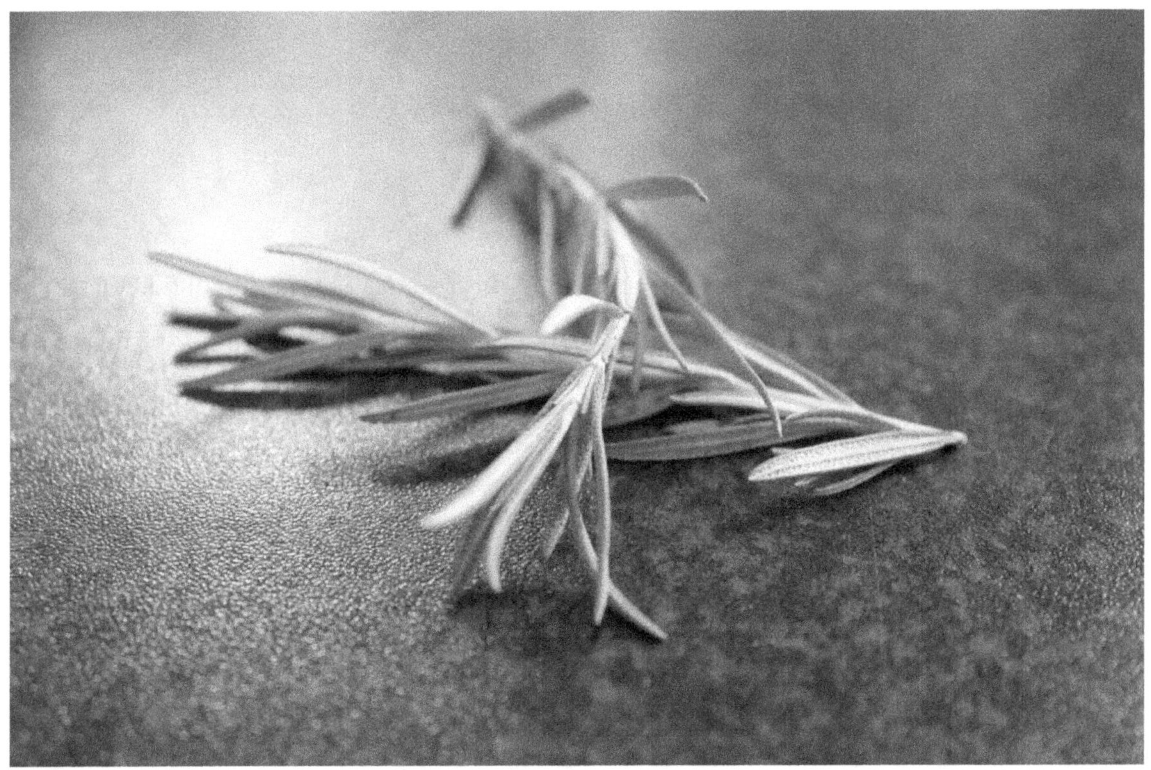

Serving Sizes: 1 Liter Jar

Prep Time: 4 hours

Ingredient List:

- Grapefruit: ½
- Rosemary: ½ sprig

XXXXXXXXXXXXXXXXXXXXXXXXXXXXXXXXXXXXXXXXXXXXXXXXXXXXXXXXXXXXX

Procedure:

Cut the skin of the grapefruit and add it to a jug. Add rosemary in the jug and keep it aside for almost 4 hours or overnight in the refrigerator. You will need a 1-liter jug.

Recipe 15: Basil and Black Tea Infusion

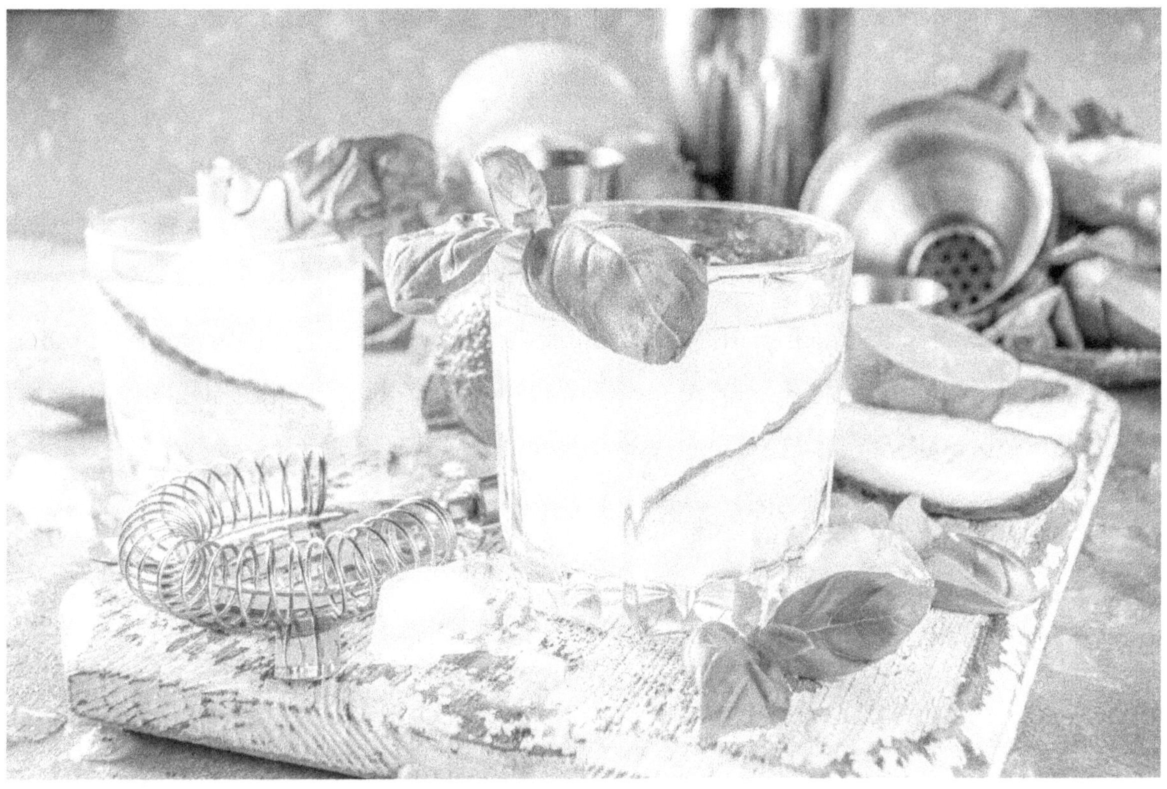

Serving Sizes: 1-liter

Prep Time: 4 hours

Ingredient List:

- Mandarin oranges: 2
- Basil leaves: 4
- Black tea bag: 1

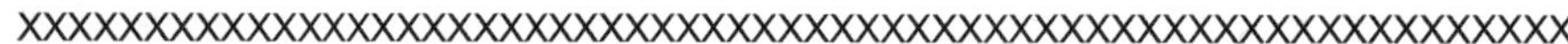

Procedure:

Peel the mandarin and slice in half. Add all ingredients to a jug filled with water. Put this jug in your room at room temperature for 4 hours or overnight and enjoy its delicious taste. This infusion is good to enhance your metabolism.

Recipe 16: Nectarine and Ginger Water

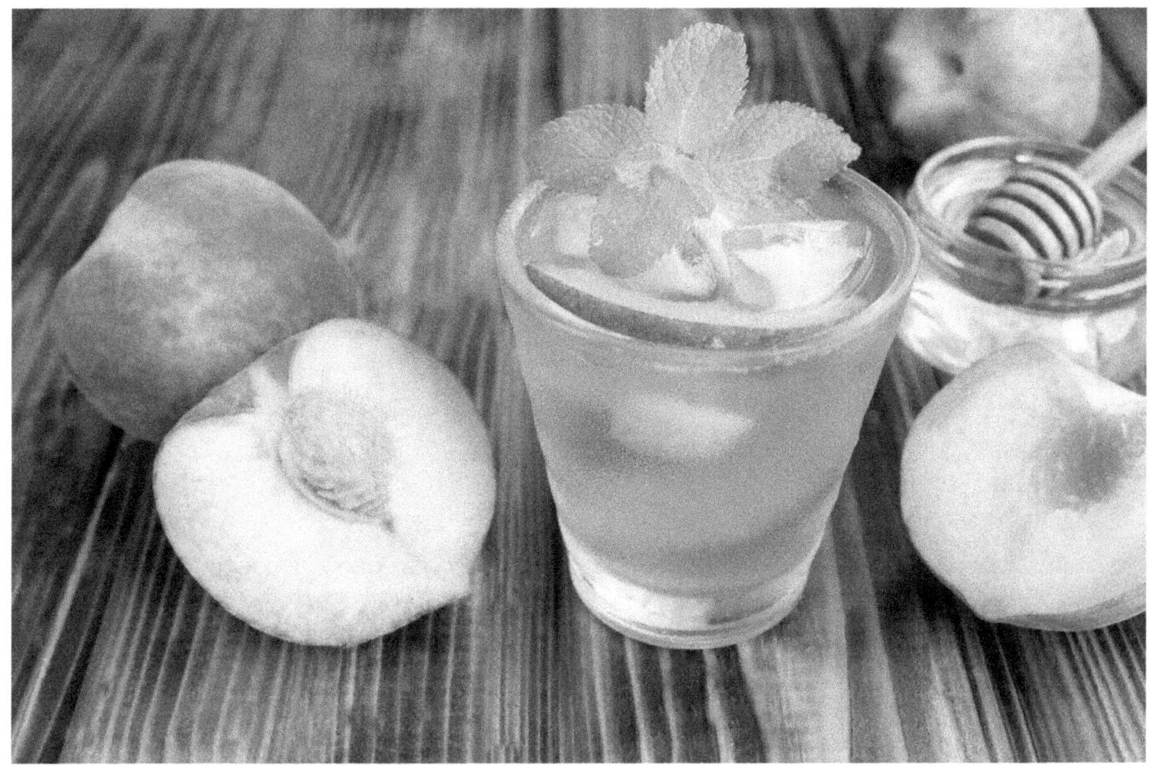

Serving Sizes: 2 quarts

Prep Time: 4 hours 15 minutes

Ingredient List:

- Lime (juiced): ½
- Thin slices of cucumber: ½ small
- Peeled ginger root: 4 slices
- Chopped and pitted nectarine: ½
- Lemon balm (Melissa leaves): 10
- Sliced lemon: ½
- Lemon juice: squeeze ½ lemon
- Sliced lime: ½
- Water: 2 quarts
- Liquid stevia: 1 drop

XXXXXXXXXXXXXXXXXXXXXXXXXXXXXXXXXXXXXXXXXXXXXXXXXXXXXXXXXXXXX

Procedure:

Put Melissa leaves, ginger, lime juice, lime slices, lemon juice, lemon slices, nectarine and cucumber in a pitcher. Use a wooden spoon to mash gently.

Pour in 2 quarts water, mix and put in the fridge for 4 hours to overnight. Strain and serve over sufficient ice.

Recipe 17: Ginger and Cinnamon Infusion

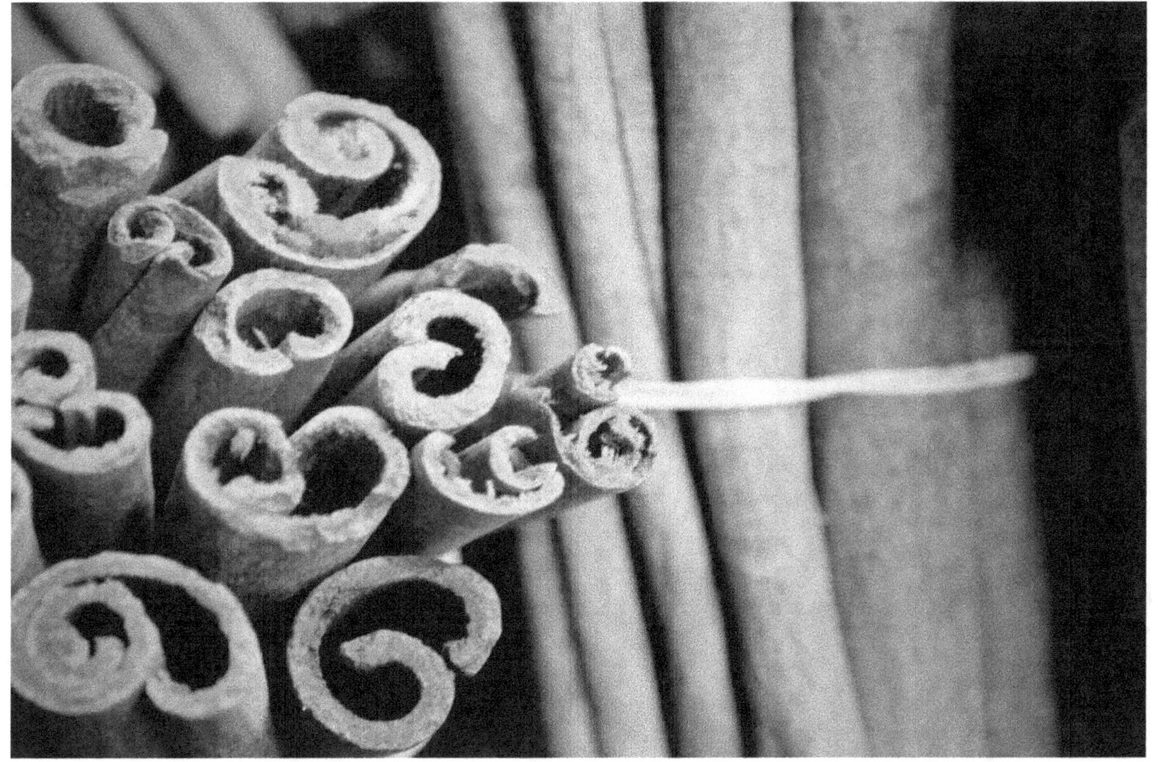

Serving Sizes: 1 gallon

Prep Time: 4 hours

Ingredient List:

- Cinnamon sticks: 2
- Lemons: 2
- Water: 1 gallon
- Fresh ginger: 3-inch piece
- Pear: 1 (elongated cuts)

XXXXXXXXXXXXXXXXXXXXXXXXXXXXXXXXXXXXXXXXXXXXXXXXXXXXXXXXXXXXXXX

Procedure:

Wash ginger and lemons. Slice lemons and pear and make thin slices of ginger. Put lemon slices, pear slices, cinnamon sticks, and ginger slices in a big pitcher.

Fill glass pitcher with clean water and put in the fridge for 4 hours or overnight. Serve chilled.

Recipe 18: Peach Orange Infusion

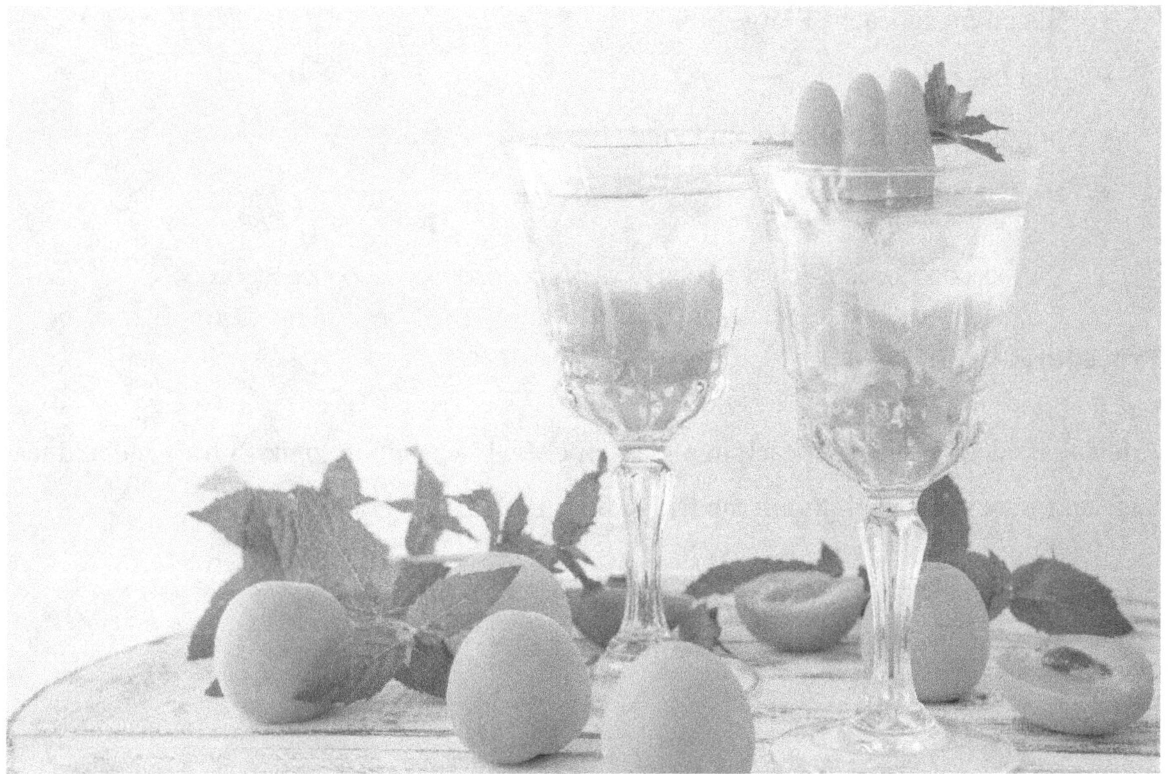

Serving Sizes: 2 liters

Prep Time: 3 hour 10 minutes

Ingredient List:

- Boiling water: 8 cups
- Sliced fresh peach: 1 large
- Tea bags: 4
- Segmented and peeled clementine: 1
- Brown sugar: 1 tbsp.

XXXXXXXXXXXXXXXXXXXXXXXXXXXXXXXXXXXXXXXXXXXXXXXXXXXXXXXXXXXXXX

Procedure:

Add sugar, clementine and peach in a glass pitcher. Use a spoon to mash fruit and add tea bags and water. Stir well. Put in the fridge for almost 2 to 3 hours.

Remove tea bags and fruit with a slotted ladle. Serve chilled.

Recipe 19: Vanilla, Mint and Lemongrass Infusion

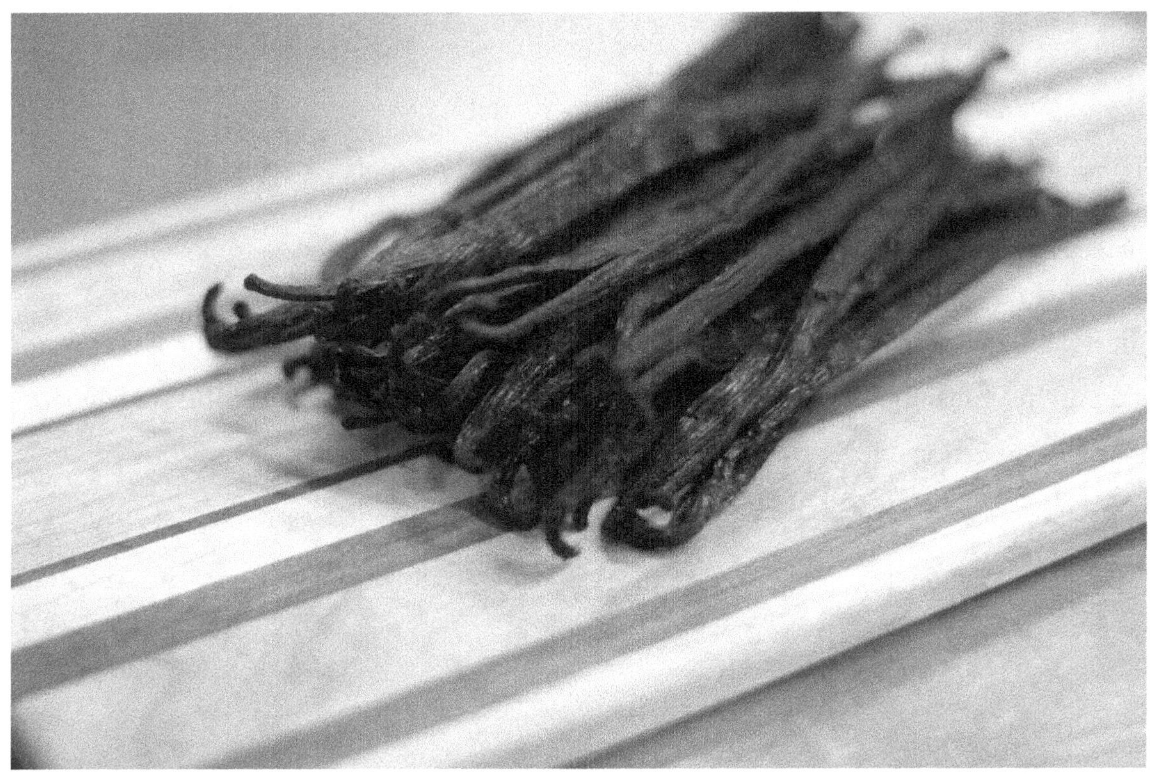

Serving Sizes: 1-liter

Prep Time: 4 hours

Ingredient List:

- Lemongrass: 1 stalk
- Mint: 2 sprigs
- Vanilla bean: 1

XXXXXXXXXXXXXXXXXXXXXXXXXXXXXXXXXXXXXXXXXXXXXXXXXXXXXXXXXXXXXXX

Procedure:

Slice vanilla bean lengthwise and add in the jug with other ingredients. Pour 1-liter water and put this infusion aside for 4 hours in the fridge. Serve chilled. This infusion is good for aches, infections, fever, respiratory disorders, insomnia, and stomach disorders.

Recipe 20: Cucumber and Tomato Water

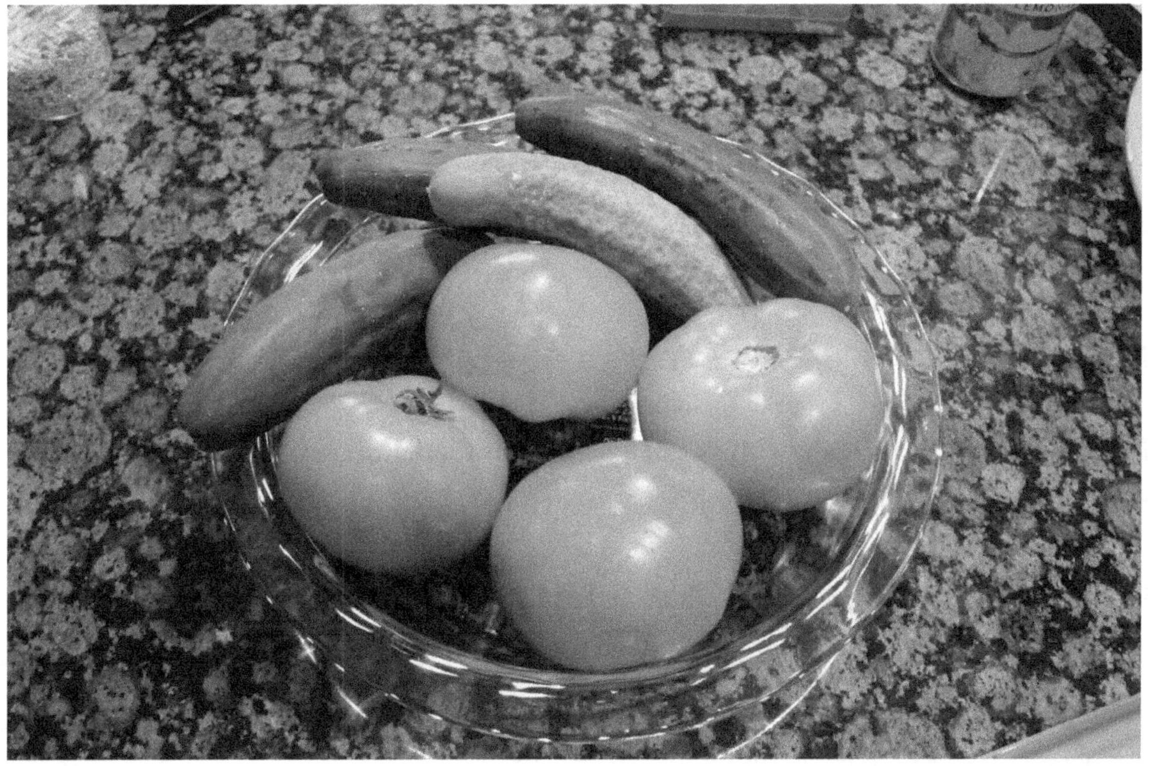

Serving Sizes: 8 cups

Prep Time: 4 hours 10 minutes

Ingredient List:

- Tomatoes (quartered, cored and stemmed): 4 pounds
- English cucumber (peeled and chopped into large chunks): 1 large
- Salt: 2 tbsp.
- Minced chives: 1 tbsp.
- Minced lemon rind: 1 tbsp.

XXXXXXXXXXXXXXXXXXXXXXXXXXXXXXXXXXXXXXXXXXXXXXXXXXXXXXXXXXX

Procedure:

Puree cucumber and tomato with salt in a blender or food processor. Line one bowl with a large cheesecloth or a clean muslin thin kitchen towel.

Pour pureed cucumber and tomato mixture in the bowl lined with towel. Gather both ends of the cheesecloth or towel and tie them to make knots. Slip one wooden spoon under and through the knot and suspend this towel over a bowl. It allows the cucumber-tomato water to slowly drip in the bowl.

Resist the impulse to squash the pulp in the cheesecloth. It can make infusion cloudy. Let the mixture drip for 4 to 8 hours and discard pulp. Put in the fridge and serve in chilled glasses or bowls with lemon rind and chives.

Recipe 21: Lavender and Blueberry Infusion

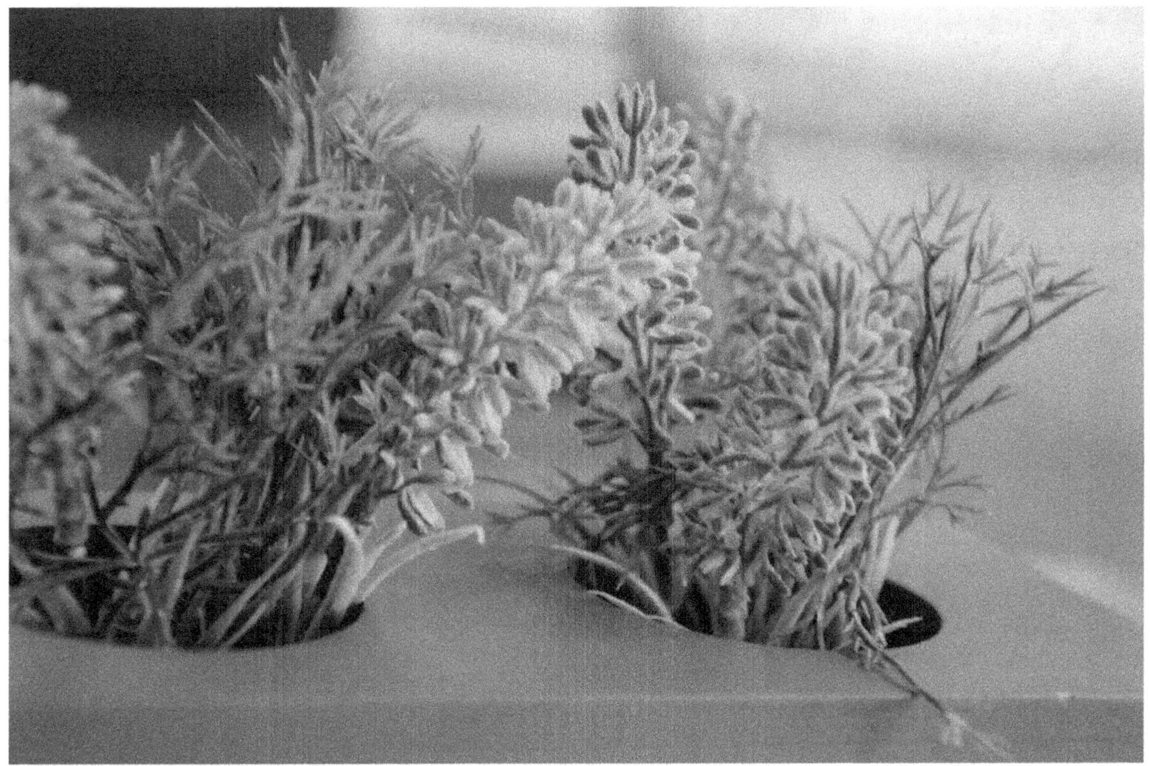

Serving Sizes: 64 ounces

Prep Time: 4 hours

Ingredient List:

- Blueberries: ½ pint
- Edible lavender flowers: to taste
- Water: 64 ounces

XXXXXXXXXXXXXXXXXXXXXXXXXXXXXXXXXXXXXXXXXXXXXXXXXXXXXXXXXXXXXX

Procedure:

Add flowers and fruits to a pitcher full of water. Cover this pitcher and chill for 4 hours. Strain and add ice. Pour in long glasses and serve.

Recipe 22: Skinny Infusion

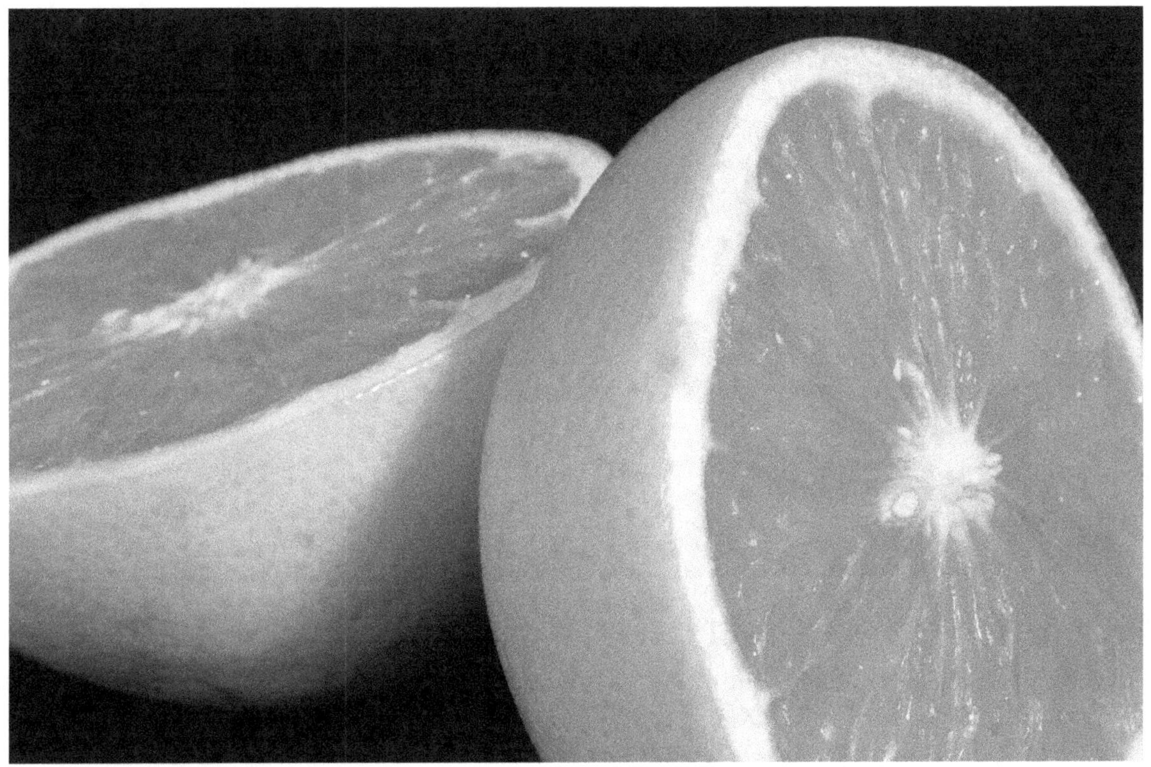

Serving Sizes: 1-liter

Prep Time: 4 hours 10 minutes

Ingredient List:

- Lemon: 4 slices
- Lime: 4 slices
- Grapefruit: 2 slices
- Cucumber: 6 slices
- Fresh Mint: 12 leaves
- Water: 1-liter
- Ice: as per need

XXXXXXXXXXXXXXXXXXXXXXXXXXXXXXXXXXXXXXXXXXXXXXXXXXXXXXXXXXXX

Procedure:

Combine ice and water in a mason jar. Add mint, cucumber, grapefruit, lime and lemon in water. Mix it for 5 minutes and put in the fridge for 4 hours or overnight to infuse flavors. It is good to enhance your metabolism and detoxify your body.

Recipe 23: Raspberry Scented Water

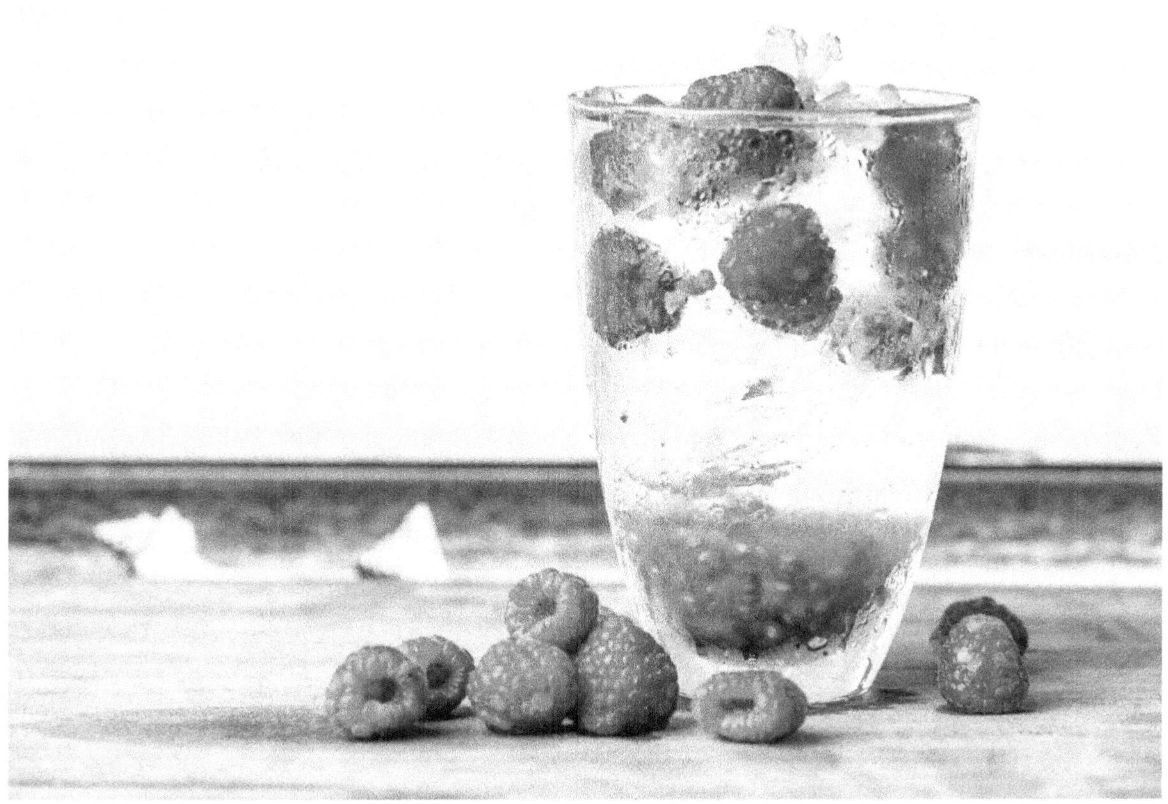

Serving Sizes: 6

Prep Time: 4 hours 15 minutes

Ingredient List:

- Filtered water or spring water: 2 liters
- Frozen or fresh raspberries: 2 tbsp.
- Mint leaves: 2 tbsp.
- Lime: 1

xxxxxxxxxxxxxxxxxxxxxxxxxxxxxxxxxxxxxxxxxxxxxxxxxxxxxxxxxxxxxx

Procedure:

Microwave lime for almost 30 seconds to get more juice and flavor. Make slices of lime.

Pour water in a jug and add lime, mint and raspberries in the jug. Stir well and keep in the fridge for 4 hours to infuse flavors. Serve chilled.

Recipe 24: Detox for Skin

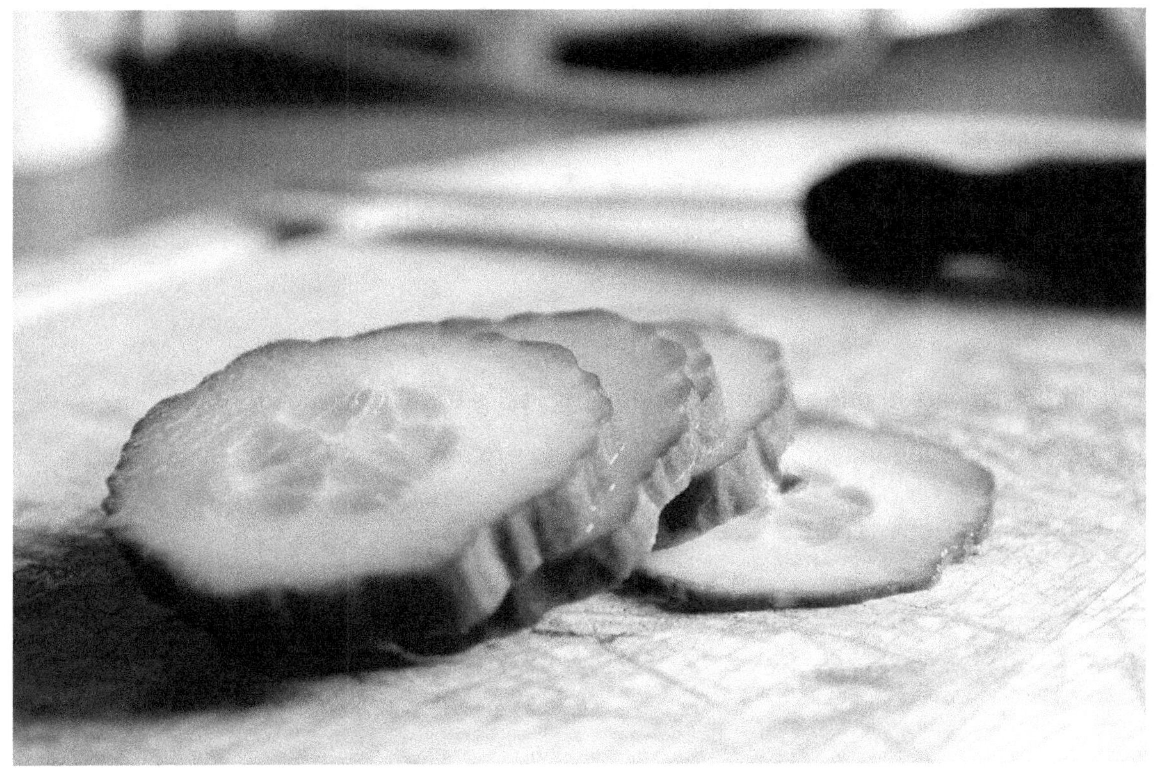

Serving Sizes: 8 cups

Prep Time: 12 hours 10 minutes

Ingredient List:

- Water: 8 cups
- Sliced or wedged cucumber: 1
- Sliced or wedged lemon: 1
- Mint leaves: 10

XXXXXXXXXXXXXXXXXXXXXXXXXXXXXXXXXXXXXXXXXXXXXXXXXXXXXXXXXXXX

Procedure:

Add all ingredients in one airtight jar and put it in the fridge for one night to infuse flavors. It will be a good choice to increase shine of your skin.

Recipe 25: Fat Burning Infused Drink

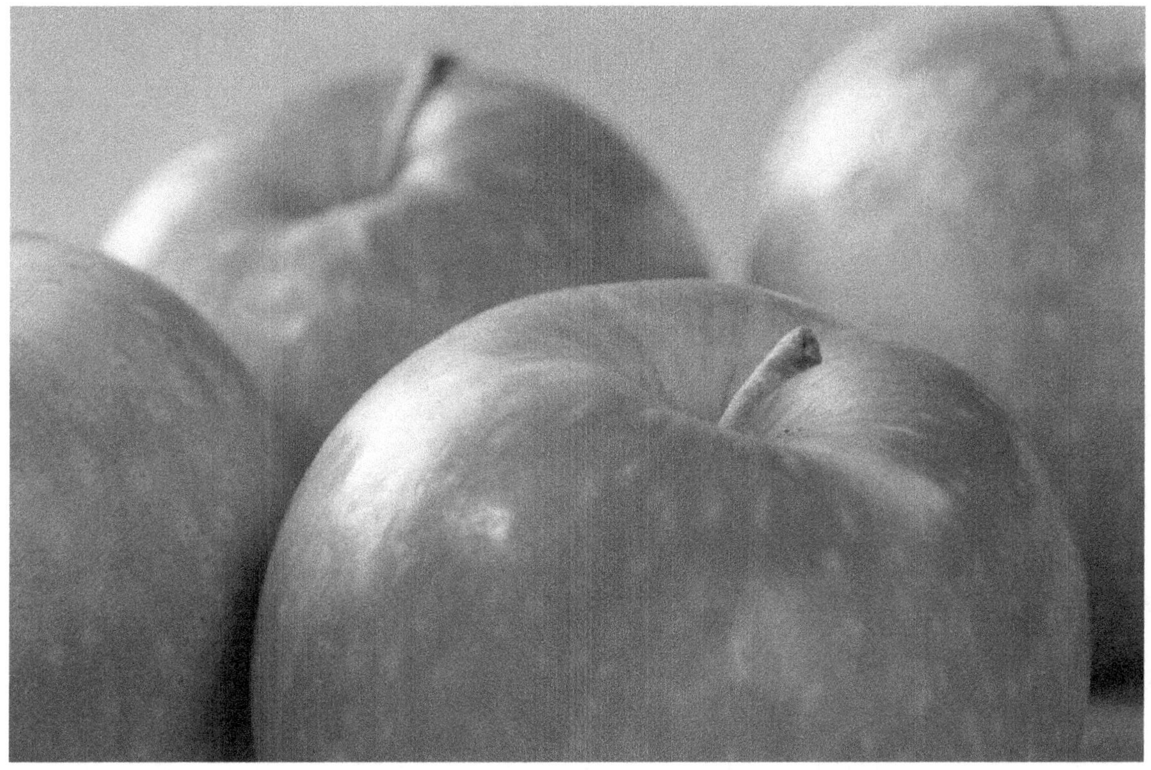

Serving Sizes: 12 ounces

Prep Time: 4 hours 10 minutes

Ingredient List:

- Water: 12 ounces
- Apple cider vinegar: 1 to 2 tbsp.
- Lemon juice: 1 tbsp.
- Cinnamon: 1 tbsp.
- Sweetener: ½ tsp.
- Apple: ½ (sliced)

XXXXXXXXXXXXXXXXXXXXXXXXXXXXXXXXXXXXXXXXXXXXXXXXXXXXXXXXXX

Procedure:

Add all ingredients (except apples) in your blender and blend for almost 10 seconds.

Add apple slices in the blend and keep it aside for almost 4 hours. Enjoy chilled. It is good to burn your extra body fat.

Author's Afterthoughts

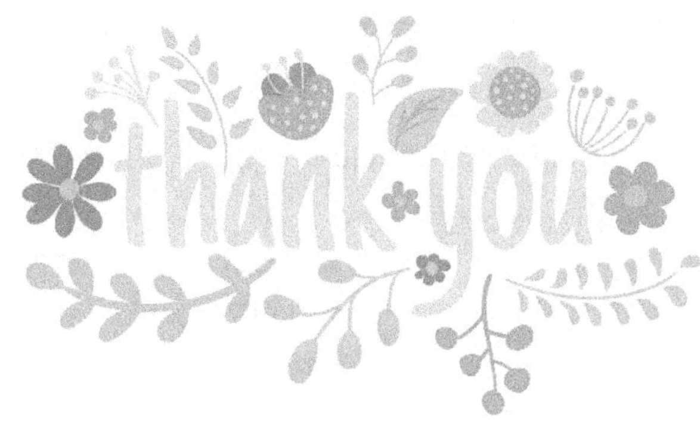

I can't appreciate you enough for spending your precious time reading my book. If there is anything that gladdens an author's heart, it is that his or her work be read. And I am extremely joyous that my labor and the hours put into making this publication a reality didn't go to waste.

Another thing that gladdens an author's heart is feedback because every comment from the good people who read one's book matters a great deal in helping you become better at what you do.

This is why I wouldn't shy away from reading your thoughts and comments about what you have read in this publication.

Do you think it is good enough? Do you think it could be better?

Please keep the feedback coming in, I won't hesitate to read any of them!!!

Thanks!

Layla Tacy

Biography

Climbing up the ladder from a young girl who loved to experiment with food items in her mother's cottage kitchen at the tender age of 7, to changing cooking from what it was to what it should be; Layla has more than made a name for herself, but she has created a dynasty for herself in the cooking world.

With more than twenty-five years in the culinary world, Layla has grown to be an authority with her influence spreading all over different high-class hotels and restaurants in and around Kansas City, such as Hilton President Kansas City, The Fountaine hotel, and Embassy Suites.

After working as a chef in different establishments, Layla moved on to become a chef-trainer to several up-and-coming chefs. Currently, she has graduated more than 200 trainees at her Chef School and presently has about 150 graduates in her school.

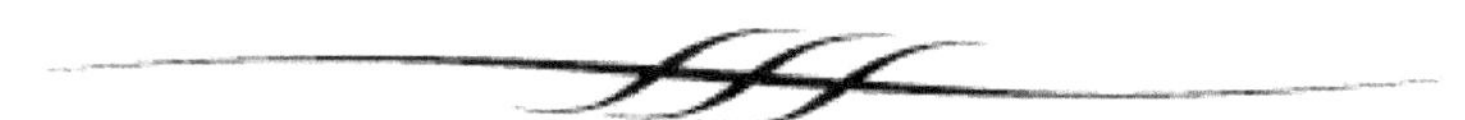

9 798761 805668